HOW TO CURE CATARRHAL DEAFNESS AND HEAD NOISES

These extremely distressing conditions evoke little sympathy for the sufferer because they exhibit no outward, visible symptoms. They are now regarded as incurable, yet the actual case histories quoted in this book prove that the author's simple self-treatment can eradicate both troubles through the application of Nature Cure methods.

By the same author
HEALING YOURSELF WITH WATER

In this series
NATURE CURE FOR HIGH BLOOD-PRESSURE
NATURE CURE FOR RHEUMATIC AILMENTS
THE NATURAL TREATMENT OF LIVER TROUBLES
THE NATURAL WAY TO SLIM SAFELY
THE NATURE CURE TREATMENT OF GASTRIC AND DUODENAL ULCERATIONS
THE NATURE CURE TREATMENT FOR VARICOSE VEINS AND ULCERS
THE SUCCESSFUL TREATMENT OF CATARRH
THE SUCCESSFUL TREATMENT OF HAIR DISORDERS

How to Cure Catarrhal Deafness and Head Noises

J. Russell Sneddon N.D., M.B.N.O.A.

THORSONS PUBLISHERS LIMITED
Wellingborough, Northamptonshire

First published 1954
Second Impression 1957
Third Impression 1963
Fourth Impression 1966
Fifth Impression 1969
Second Edition, revised and reset, 1973
Second Impression 1975
Third Impression 1978
Fourth Impression 1981

ISBN 0 7225 0221 4

Printed and bound in Great Britain by
Richard Clay (The Chaucer Press) Ltd.,
Bungay, Suffolk.

Introduction

THIS BOOK HAS been written to supply a long-felt want because it is on a subject that is very seldom treated in writings for the layman. For many years now our health has been in the hands of the medical profession, and they have always demanded that the patient must follow their advice without question. It has been the custom for each doctor to present himself as a small font of wisdom; if a disease defeated him recourse was made to the great hospitals, and if the disease was still the victor there the patient was deemed incurable.

In all the various situations in which the patient found himself he was never treated as a thinking being, but rather as some sort of imbecile, who could not understand treatment in any form, even if it were explained very simply. As a result of this, people gradually came to think about health as something that could only be gained by strict obedience to the laws of the medicine man.

Even today there are many millions of people who do not understand that health is natural and that it is the giving of medicines that is the unnatural part of the whole business. Man is not built to live in ill-health but in health, and everything has been arranged by nature to enable that happy state to be reached.

In this modern age we have much to increase the chances of a long healthy life, with better conditions of work and play, with more leisure, greater creative powers and many hobbies which bring about that relaxation of the mind which is essential to its vitality.

With the advent of sanitary engineering, perhaps the greatest step towards health has been taken during the last fifty years, resulting in the removal of the conditions that brought about a rapid growth of destructive bacteria. All the essentials to a life of health and abundance are now present, but there are two factors that still prevent us from obtaining the full benefit of this progress.

The first is that the medical profession refuses to take responsibility for supplying fresh, wholesome food to the people. By this is meant food that is tasteful and appetizing and meets all the requirements needed for health. It also means that such food should not give rise to end-results that are detrimental to the body in any way. Are these conditions now fulfilled? By no means!

SHAM FOODS

Every thinking person knows that most foodstuffs are cleansed until they are useless, sterilized, pasteurized and dyed until, although they may have some advertising value, they are mere shams of their natural state. In addition to these changes, synthetic flavours, colouring matter, fillers and fat sparers are introduced – all substances that may or may not do harm to the body. The reactions of these substances within the body are unknown, but the many peculiar symptoms now manifest make them very suspect.

Mineral salts taken from the flour during milling are reintroduced in another form, and in such a way that the impression is given that the flour is better than the original devised by nature.

Many of these changes which are allowed to take place in our food are definitely injurious to our health, and in this time of abundance, when all the modern discoveries could be turned to help man, there is still a great lack of action on the part of our medical advisers.

The second factor that prevents us from taking full advantage of progress is the increase in the number of drugs used in cases of ill-health. Everything that enters the mouth should be, strictly speaking, a food or liquid that will be of benefit to the body. In a modern world such as ours – a chemicalized world, it could be termed – this is difficult, because nearly everything is tampered with in some way. Yet the doctor can again be taken to task because he is giving medicines, of which he knows little except perhaps the chemical formula, in ever-increasing amounts. We are fast becoming a nation of drug-takers!

MEDICINES ARE SUSPECT

The reaction of one drug within one body may be totally different from the reaction of the same drug within another body. This is often found, and when detrimental effects arise the patient is glibly told that he or she is allergic to that drug and that it should not be taken. The allergy only shows one reaction. A person may be adversely affected by a drug, may suffer severely from it, yet the reaction may be very slow and only appear months or years afterwards; and when it does occur it is treated as a symptom of some new disease. Medicines, whether they are modern or old-fashioned, are not foods and must always be suspect. Whether introduced orally or given in the form of injection, they can be dangerous, and they are so because they are unnatural to our bodies.

So the medical man does not subscribe to health in two main ways. First of all, he allows our food to be adulterated; and, as the body is built on food, this is the main source of modern ill-health. Secondly, instead of teaching the people how to live naturally, he is subscribing more and more to the general idea that health can be obtained from medicines. The amount of drugs consumed in this country is now reaching a tremendous figure, and special hospitals are being built to deal with the ever-increasing number of drug addicts.

CYCLE OF ILL-HEALTH

There are some people who argue that ill-health springs from badly fed soil and maintain that our fruit, vegetables and grains are in a state of unbalance because much of our soil is over-worked and fed only by artificial manures. These in turn supply unnatural substances which are received into the vegetables, grains and fruits, and so unbalance them. They also maintain that all animals fed on poor land become ill, and that these animals cannot give healthy produce. It is easy to follow that if the animals themselves are unhealthy, than the manure from them cannot be healthy. Thus we have a very serious cycle of ill-health.

This problem of the soil is vital and needs thorough investigation. The people who cultivate and rest their land according to natural laws make great claims, and these cannot long be denied. For instance, they maintain that foot-and-mouth disease, so common in animals in all countries, but especially in Europe, does not affect animals fed on ground that has been naturally composted and manured. Indeed, it is maintained that these animals can be placed in actual physical contact with animals suffering from this very virulent trouble without being affected in any way.

This is a very great challenge, and it is of interest to all of us, not only for health but also from the point of view of finance, because all the great losses caused by foot-and-mouth disease have to be borne by the taxpayer. Thousands and thousands of pounds are lost with each outbreak, because all animals affected or that have been in contact with affected animals are immediately destroyed. The claims for compensation are large; and if the above contention is true this tremendous loss to the country can be avoided.

The growers of vegetables, fruits and cereals have a duty to the community. That duty is that the food which they sell should be fresh and healthy. Yet this is not always the case. Indeed, we are now getting to the stage that it is very seldom the case, because vegetables and fruits now obtainable are usually subjected to much chemicalization before reaching the shops.

DRUGLESS HEALING

Talking about food naturally leads to the methods of arranging meals to suit the various states of ill-health. The people who study this technique are called dietitians, and they can be divided into two main classes, medical and non-medical. Naturally those trained in a medical atmosphere absorb the teachings of doctors. The methods of diet outlined in this book are non-medical and based on Nature Cure. They are the results of findings extending over many years of dieting, because Nature Cure practitioners have always been interested in diet and are specialists in the art of using food for healing purposes.

In this age another aspect of the findings of the pioneer naturopaths is coming under the spotlight of modern medicine. It is now called the study of 'body mechanics,' and simply means ensuring that every organ of the body is in its proper position and that the spine has its proper curves. This has always been studied by Nature Cure practitioners and osteopathic practitioners, and this study is included in all methods of cure.

With these points in mind, this book has been written for sufferers from catarrhal deafness and head noises. Herein is described a drugless method of healing, based on good wholesome food and the obeying of the dictates of natural law.

Contents

Chapter		*Page*
1.	Causes	13
2.	The Curative Fast	18
3.	Vegetables and Acid Fruits	24
4.	Food Factors	29
5.	The Diet	34
6.	Elimination	41
7.	Local Treatment	47
8.	Some Cures	54
9.	Head Noises	60

I.
Causes

THE TYPE OF deafness we are studying, that of catarrhal origin, is not so serious as nerve deafness. The latter is practically incurable, except in certain cases where a good result can be obtained by complicated and dangerous surgical operations. The cattarrhal type of deafness, however, is insidious, progressive, and, if accompanied by head noises, gradually assumes the proportion of a major trouble. It usually starts in childhood and is associated with a general catarrhal tendency and enlarged tonsils and adenoids. These latter glandular substances have a particular function in the body: to prevent the entrance into the system, through the nose and mouth, of germs that would be detrimental to the body. They form part of a cycle of glands which are protective in their mechanism, and this must be remembered before we allow surgical removal of the parts.

THE PROTECTIVE RING

In childhood, frequent bouts of inflammation in these glands are often accompanied by transient deafness, and the general medical advice is to have the adenoids and tonsils surgically removed. Whenever this is done, the protective ring, the guarding mechanism of the body, is broken, and it will have some detrimental effect on the health of the person at some later date. It cannot be denied that the surgical removal of these glands improves catarrhal deafness in many cases. In others it makes no difference whatsoever, and the deafness is allowed to proceed unchecked. When, however, relief can be obtained by removing the catarrhal cause without breaking this protective circle, then we are getting much closer to the real treatment of this trouble. Deafness in children must never be regarded as an incurable complaint, but rather as a sign that a general treatment for catarrh is necessary.

In this book, therefore, it will be assumed that the real cause of deafness does not lie in the swollen tonsils and adenoids of the sufferer, but deeper, much deeper in the system. It is at this level that the real cause will be found.

There is one common factor in this trouble, and that is poor tissue drainage. It is present in every person who suffers from catarrhal deafness. This is a positive finding which has been noted in the investigations of many practitioners. A short explanation is needed to explain what is actually meant by this finding.

Around all the tissues of the body there flows a fluid called the 'lymph.' Its purpose is to supply a means of drainage for the tissues and ease of removal of impurities that occur in the normal working of each cell. Lymph is also used as a method of conveying to the tissues the foods and salts essential to their health.

When this lymphatic fluid is working normally, the debris of combustion and of the various usages of the cells is easily excreted, and the cells are supplied with food – provided, of course, that food is introduced in the diet. When, however, the lymphatic fluid is sluggish, then the cells become congested and the tissue naturally enlarges and a state of inflammation may arise. Any impurity that is free within the circulation tends to collect where congestion is found, and such a collection often arises in the neck area.

POOR CIRCULATION

This storing of impurity, within a near radius of the ear, is the main factor of catarrhal deafness. The primary cause, however, is the deficient lymphatic circulation, and the people who suffer from it generally have poor blood circulation. This means that the blood does not flow rapidly enough through the system, especially in the extremities. These people have cold hands and feet and generally feel the cold weather intensely.

The question now is, what brings about poor lymphatic circulation? To a large extent there are hereditary tendencies, but in most cases the cause lies in the poor choice of food and lack of body hygiene.

That hereditary influence plays a great part in the condition of the lymphatic circulation cannot be denied, and it will often be found that the weakness of one parent, especially a parent who tends to deafness, is given to all offspring. This weakness, that of poor circulation in the tissues, does not always mean that the person suffers from a weak general circulation. The defect is only in the lymphatic system, and as age increases, more and more congestion appears, and with it some irritation that may cause head noises. If an increased circulation of the lymphatic stream in the ear and adjacent tissues can be achieved, then much has been done to eradicate the cause of catarrhal deafness.

Although certain lymphatic tendencies pass down from a parent to a child, and even through several generations, there is another factor of great importance. It is that the original cause of the lymphatic weakness has never been treated. Yet this can be corrected by choice of food and by abstinence from certain liquids and the study of food rules; in short, by measures that increase the circulation.

In doing so a vicious cycle is broken. There is a general tendency for the offspring to be fed in a very similar manner to the parents, and this form of feeding is carried from one generation to another. Certain foods and liquids that are definitely harmful, and which were taken by the forebears of the person suffering from catarrhal deafness, are also taken by the person now suffering from deafness; that is, the general food tendency of a family is very much the same throughout several generations. In our efforts to find the cure of catarrhal deafness and head noises it will often be our duty to break up this sequence. We must do so if we are to achieve the desired result, that is, the curing and prevention of catarrhal deafness and head noises.

LESION IN NECK BONES

There is another circulation, or really another part of the lymphatic circulation, which must also be stimulated if a cure is to be achieved. Osteopaths – that is, practitioners who make a study of the bones and the effects of misalignment on the nervous system – have made valuable discoveries. They have found that lesions or displacements of the bones of the neck can bring about poor lymphatic circulation in the tissues around the ears. This is a vital finding, and it gives a clue to the reason why one person becomes deaf and another person, living practically in the same circumstances, is not affected. In other words, two people in the same family may have hereditary catarrhal weaknesses, but one is affected by deafness and the other is not. The main reason for this distinction is some form of lesion in the neck bones. Such a lesion can be brought about by a childhood fall, a blow on the head, indeed any fairly slight accident that may pass without apparent ill-effect. In many cases it is difficult to find when a particular lesion was sustained, although a practitioner can often obtain a clue by deducing the duration of the trouble.

The reader may wonder how such a lesion can be cured. It must be understood that if there is a lesion of the neck bones, professional osteopathic treatment is the best way to obtain correction. In this book, however, although the benefits of the professional treatment are stressed, we will give other methods of relieving tissue impingement. Please note that tissue, not nerve impingement, is mentioned. It is seldom that the nerve is directly affected. Tension, created in the muscles and ligaments by the lesion, is usually reflected upon the nerves and brings about disturbances of the circulation controlled by these nerves. In other words, if we can exercise by specific movements of groups of muscles, the nerve pressure can be relieved and often the bony lesions will adjust themselves during the performing of the exercises. If, however, a very severe lesion is suspected, say in a case in which a severe fall has resulted in some form of deafness, then the services of a fully trained naturopath should be sought, because in this instance a definite manipulative technique is required.

In the large majority of cases the exercising of the neck muscles and ligaments, systematically performed, will bring about the release of most of the general tension, and in doing so will remove the irritation that is often affecting the ear. This is a most important point and should allay the fears of any reader who considers he must have professional manipulation as quickly as possible.

We can now divide the causes of catarrhal deafness and head noises into two main classifications. First, the primary cause is poor lymphatic circulation, which creates some congestion of the tissues of the body, and, in particular, of the tissues around the ear. Secondly, some lesion of the spine or some impingement caused by any factor makes the lymphatic circulation more inefficient in the area of the ear. With these two main factors in mind, we can now go ahead and study how they can be corrected.

2.
The Curative Fast

OUR FIRST TASK must be to increase the speed of lymphatic flow. It has been the finding of many practitioners, interested in diet, that certain foodstuffs and certain liquids introduce materials into the body that slow the lymphatic flow, and these foods and liquids must be eliminated from the diet to bring about a cure. This naturally takes time, and it is not possible immediately to stop the intake of the harmful materials; indeed, it is not wise to make rapid changes in the diet at all, because the healing forces of the body may be so stirred that they bring about a vigorous reaction within a few weeks. So we must tackle this problem in a logical manner, making one change after another and gradually building a diet and system of eating that accomplishes our aim, which is to increase the drainage of the body through the lymphatic stream.

Steps to set the cure into action, however, can be immediate because it has been found that when the body is fasted a great deal of the impurity lying in the tissues is set free in the circulation. This may be due to the fact that the body gets a rest during a fast. No energy has to be dissipated in digestion, and the body immediately takes advantage of this to clear some of the congested organs. Experiments have proved that even large masses of congestion, masses that could be termed 'tumours,' are removed by the simple process of fasting. So start the treatment immediately by having two days' fast. This means that nothing but water is taken, and this is definitely the best type of fasting.

There are many forms of fasting – plain fasting on water,

fasting on fruit or vegetable juice – but the most effective and perhaps the one that can be conducted by everyone is the plain fast already advised. If the reader has no experience of fasting it would be advisable to understand actually what takes place.

CLEANSING SIGNS

Whenever the body is deprived of food but given liquid, there is a great deal of cleansing undertaken in the digestive system. As a result the tongue becomes coated and thickened, and often the patient becomes very thirsty. In this case, of course, water can be taken to allay the thirst. Headaches, especially of a frontal nature, are also common. There is normally a great desire to eat something, but this usually can be withstood at least for a day or two, if the patient is fully aware of what he or she is attempting to cure.

At night, even after a day's fasting, in addition to the pangs of hunger, the patient will be aware of a certain restlessness and general disturbance. If the fast is carried over the next day it will usually be found there is a headache on rising and the tongue will be in a fairly dirty condition. These are quite normal sensations and show that the fast is doing what is desired – that is, bringing about a cleansing of the digestive system.

With one or two days' fast, if the patient can manage it, the first stage has been taken in overcoming catarrhal deafness. A start has been made on drawing the impurities away from the congested areas. They were congested because too much catarrhal material was introduced into the body, and finally the lymphatics were unable to deal with this excess. So, before we go on to the study of the more minute aspects of diet, I would advise all sufferers to begin the treatment with two days on nothing but water. If it is desired that fruit juice be taken, then apple, orange or grapefruit juice is allowed. These actually are vital substances in that they stimulate the cleansing properties of the body, and there is more disturbance in the system than with the ordinary fast on water. The fruit-juice fast is more suitable for the young and vigorous patient.

In some cases fruit juice causes acidity of the stomach, and this is one factor against this type of fast. It should not be undertaken by anyone who has any history of digestive ailment such as gastritis or gastric-duodenal ulcers. The acid introduced in the fruit juice will disturb these parts and may cause quite a digestive upset.

WASHING OUT THE BOWEL

With the fast goes the enema, and it is always advisable after a two-day fast to wash out the bowel. If the fast is continued during the second day, I rather favour the taking of quite a considerable amount of water on the second day – say, four to six pints – because this gives the body an internal bath and aids in the cleansing of the digestive tract. It must not be thought that all the impurities that come from the digestive tract were actually lying there before the fast, because it has been found that the body will remove impurity from other parts of the system and deliver this impurity at the digestive tube, using the digestive part of the system as an eliminative organ. When a two-day fast has been undertaken it is advisable to wash out the bowel at the end of the second day. This is best done by using the warm-water enema.

The best type of enema is the can type, which holds from two to four pints of water and is placed about four or five feet from the floor. This can is filled with two or three pints of water, which is comfortably warm, and the nozzle end, first of all greased with vaseline, is gently inserted into the rectum, usually when the patient is lying on his right side. When the nozzle has been inserted as far as it can be without discomfort, the small valve at the end is opened and the warm water is allowed to flow gently into the bowel. This may cause a little discomfort at the beginning, and for a few seconds the water may require to be shut off and then released again and more water allowed to pass into the rectum. In this way it is possible to introduce three or even four pints of water in the descending part of the large bowel and rectum. Once the water has entered, the nozzle should be carefully withdrawn and the patient should lie on his back, then on his right side, retaining the water as long as possible. When the desire to void the contents of the bowel is very strong, the water should then be allowed to come away.

If this enema is taken at the end of the second day and in conjunction with the large amount of water which has been advised as a drink, then a great deal of cleansing of the whole digestive tract will be appreciated, and, without doubt, a large amount of catarrhal material will have been removed. Taking an enema appears to be a much more difficult performance than it actually is because its description makes it appear a rather fearsome business.

TWO-DAY FAST AIDS HEARING

It will be noticed that I have not advised the enema after one day's fast. This time is too limited to bring about a good cleansing, and at least two days on nothing but water are required to get a beneficial result. The reader will be anxious to know when this type of fasting should be performed. At the beginning of the treatment is best, and, especially if a person is underweight or very much overweight, one day's fast may be taken once weekly with every benefit. If, however, it is decided that a two-day fast would be more advantageous, this should be taken every fourteen days. It will result in a very much cleaner system; indeed, it is the experience of many people suffering from catarrhal deafness that after the two-day fast they are hearing better, and this shows the great healing that attends this system of cleansing. Usually, however, a beginner in dieting finds difficulty in completing a two-day fast.

During fasting of such short duration there is no need to make any other change in the system of of living. It is quite possible to do hard physical work while fasting for two days. The fast rather invigorates and increases the working powers, and it is only when the fast is prolonged, say to fourteen days or longer, that the person requires to increase the amount of rest. If it is decided to have fruit instead of the plain warm-water fast, then it will usually be advisable to wash out the bowel each night – that is, at the end of each day's fasting.

At this stage of the treatment I am not inclined to advise any prolonged fasting. This type of treatment is most helpful when the body has been treated over a period of months by a good diet and by the other measures included in this book. Then it may be required to fast for two, three, four or even more days to stimulate the reaction and bring about the removal of very severe catarrhal congestion in the ears. This, however, is not common, and the treatment advised is usually sufficient to bring about a slow but progressive improvement in the condition of the hearing.

HEAD NOISES

It is often found that the hearing improves considerably before there is any lessening of the head noises. Head noises, usually caused by some catarrhal impingement along the nerve route of the internal ear or even against the drum itself, are always difficult to remove. Usually there is no sudden cessation; the improvement is gradual, and the head noises become less noticeable to the patient. Readers must appreciate that everything about this cure is gradual and they must not expect quick results, therefore they must not be disappointed if there is no improvement in hearing or in the cessation of head noises within a short time.

Many years have passed in the formation of the catarrhal state which leads to deafness and head noises, and this must be appreciated by the sufferer. Such complaints do not arise quickly unless as the result of a severe accident. They come gradually over a period, not of months, but of years, and the actual dullness of hearing and the sensation of head noise is the end of a chain of circumstances – a chain that is leading the patient into a state of lymphatic congestion; and it is impossible to start a cure in the final stage and bring about a rapid result. We must retrace our footsteps over the years. But it is possible by fasting, and often by increasing the severity of the treatment, to bring about a fairly quick result.

The patient who is young and vigorous can increase the intensity of treatment by fasting frequently and using various other methods that increase the cleansing effort. Owing to the very nature of the illness, however, the catarrhal deaf person is not usually very vigorous. There has been a slowing down over a period of years of the vigorous tendencies, and it is unlikely that, at least at the commencement of the treatment, severe measures will be helpful.

As the weeks pass into months, however, a certain degree of invigoration will be recognized by the person who follows this cure. This feeling of well-being should increase the intensity of the cure. He should fast, he should fruit-fast, he should do more exercises, he should get out in the open air, he should walk, he should deep-breathe, he should avoid all the debilitating habits, and his reward will be great; it will also come very much more quickly than that of the person who is physically incapable of making a greater effort. This can be followed, of course, quite easily. It is the natural thing, and the person who is not physically capable of bringing about a rapid cure must be content to follow out the actions explained in this book as carefully as possible, reading each chapter and understanding the meaning of each idea as it is presented to him. Then he will build up a mind picture of how he can progress towards health.

3.
Vegetables and Acid Fruits

A HEALTH-GIVING diet must be based on certain principles. The first is to introduce food that gives everything the body requires to sustain the necessary heat and energy and supply the mineral salts and vitamins required for health. Secondly, the food must contain eliminative factors, that is, substances that aid the removal of the end-results of digestion and cell usage and prevent the accumulation within the tissues of debris and impurities which, if retained, are harmful.

The diet outlined in this book is based mainly on elimination. This is deliberate, because most of the people who need this diet are or have been in ill-health, and the cure for every disease must start with elimination. Naturally, as progress is made, a more full diet can be taken, but at first the main idea should be to cleanse the system.

To ensure complete elimination it is necessary that a sufficiency of mineral salts be taken daily. These are obtained from vegetables, and at the beginning of this book it was stressed that vegetables can be taken freely if they are grown on healthy soil. It is still difficult to obtain such vegetables, but some growers are making a determined effort to supply them. These people must be supported whenever possible, and the sufferer from catarrhal deafness, undertaking this diet, should find where these healthy vegetables can be obtained. Home-grown vegetables are, of course, the ideal, because the condition of the soil can be regulated and the vitamin content is very high if the vegetables are taken straight from the soil to the table.

It is useless continually to eat vegetables that by themselves are not high-quality foods, and such is the state of our food today that we must seek it in balanced form rather than be content with anything that is delivered to us. Vegetables, compost grown, are the basis of this treatment, for they supply mineral salts that have already been built into the vegetable from the soil. These salts can be utilized by our bodies to bring about the various chemical changes essential to elimination and health.

RAW VEGETABLES BEST

Vegetables are best taken raw and, contrary to the general belief, if they are thoroughly masticated in the raw state it will be found that they will give a much higher percentage of health factors than when steamed or conservatively cooked. Many people believe that raw vegetables are indigestible and give rise to a great deal of flatulence. This is completely wrong. They do not cause great digestive upset if completely masticated. It is surprising to find in practice that many people suffering from a severe digestive ailment, such as gastric ulcer, can digest raw vegetables and utilize them to the full without any discomfort. The same people often suffer great pain on eating cooked vegetables.

This is all against what we have been taught, but it is the finding of experienced practitioners, and, except for the rare instances in which the hard edges of the vegetables cause pain by irritation, it will generally be found that raw vegetables can be taken in nearly any condition. Certainly there is always a particular vegetable to which a patient is allergic. These tendencies vary with the individual and can only be discovered by personal experience, but I wish to emphasise that as a health-giver the vegetable is very much in advance of the fruit. It contains a larger proportion of mineral salts and, if fresh, supplies useful vitamins.

Every patient suffering from catarrhal deafness and head noises must become fully acquainted with this finding, and whenever wholesome vegetables are obtainable they should be included in the diet at least twice daily. Some people prefer to take them raw at both these meals in the form of a salad.

Other people prefer to take vegetables cooked at one meal and raw at another. Two raw vegetable salads are preferable to a steamed vegetable meal and a raw salad, but, of course, this is largely a matter of taste.

Anyone who studies dietetics is acquainted with the rule that the acid fruits turn alkaline in the stomach and give an alkaline reaction during the remainder of their passage down the digestive tract. This is only partially true, and in actual practice it is found that to many people the taking of the acid fruits results in some form of digestive acidity. It appears that in these people the alkaline elements are lacking. These are obtained from vegetables and whole-wheat products, and this is another reason why the intake of vegetables is so important. Vegetables are the basic substances, the foundation upon which the diet is built.

MINERAL SALTS

It is possible to quote instances of very healthy people who have never eaten vegetables. These people have received at birth what can be called an amount of residual mineral salts. Whether this amount is stored in their bones or is available only on certain occasions is difficult to discover, but they are able to draw, from some source within their body, the salts and minerals necessary to maintain health. The exception proves the rule. Most of us introduce mineral salts practically daily into our bodies, and if they are omitted our digestion suffers and then fruits of the acid type tend to cause acidity.

It is usually better to begin dieting by increasing the amount of vegetables (especially raw), to enable the supply of mineral salts, especially those of an alkaline nature, to be built up. These salts definitely allow the body to make much more use of other foods and liquids than if a diet is immediately started by making a complete change of food of every kind.

Both the acid and the dried fruits have their place in the diet of a person suffering from catarrh of the hearing apparatus. The acid fruits – mainly apples, oranges, grapefruit, pineapple, lemons and certain forms of berries – are very useful cleansing foods, and they are normally included in the diet with the specific purpose of stimulating the lymphatic drainage and increasing the powers of elimination. By themselves they have little food value, and they act mainly as vitalizers and suppliers of vitamins. They also contain a certain amount of mineral salts.

ACID FRUIT INTAKE ESSENTIAL

It is as cleansers, however, stimulators of elimination, that the acid fruits are of most value, and they are helpful to all who suffer from poor circulation in the lymphatic tissues. Experimentation with the acid fruits is essential, because one person will find that a certain fruit agrees with him and yet another finds that it wildly disagress. Many peculiar findings occur in the acid fruit study, and each person requires to built a diet that will contain at least one acid fruit each day and preferably two or three. These fruits add to the eliminative tendencies of the body, supplying minerals and vitamins, but they should not cause any acidity or bring about any peculiar symptoms. In other words, if an acid gives rise to skin outbreak, mouth ulceration, indigestion or like symptoms, then that fruit should be stopped, because it is not being utilized beneficially. It may be helpful, but the body is in no state to use it, and another period on vegetables and vegetable juice may be required before this fruit can be used advantageously by the body.

Acid fruit should therefore be taken as freely as possible, after an initial period on vegetables, provided there are no ill-effects. This is one golden rule. The second is that it must be taken only at the meal prescribed in the diet sheet and not at any other time. If more fruit is required the best time is between meals, away from all other foods. This is advised because acid fruit is difficult to digest and requires to be combined with certain specified foods to prevent digestive disturbance.

It will be seen in the food chart that the acid fruits are advised only with one meal, that is, the protein meal because experience has proved that they do not combine well with the starchy foods. They help in the digestion of the protein foods and enable the body to deal quickly and completely with them.

Ensuring that the acid fruits are taken in their correct food combination is a most important point and should be thoroughly studied. In many instances it will be found that a meal with an acid fruit dessert is often seemingly incomplete, and the person rises from the table feeling that the meal has not been satisfying. This is a common finding, but it will usually disappear after a few weeks' dieting, as the bowel will then be able to deal more fully with the fruit dessert.

4. Food Factors

MOST PEOPLE SUFFERING from catarrhal deafness have a rather unclean bowel, and have reached the stage in which only certain foods are digested and assimilated. These foods are mainly of the starchy, milky nature, and it is these that are the primary cause of this ailment. The catarrhal sufferer has, over a period of years, allowed the bowel to become so inactive that the difficult foods, digestively – namely the acid fruits, vegetables, proteins and whole grains – are left very much alone and pass through the bowel mainly untouched by the digestive juices. It is this very factor that leads to the unbalancing of the food supply to the actual tissues of the body. Many people eat a considerable amount of food and still starve their bodies because of their poor assimilative capacity.

Fruit and vegetables are difficult foods to digest, but they can be assimilated if the digestive tract is re-educated, and this is one of the basic factors of this treatment.

It will now be understood that this is a whole treatment, not concerned with giving any specific cure for a certain complaint, but actually cleansing the body internally and allowing it to utilize its assimilative powers to the full. All assimilation practically takes place in the small bowel, and here a rather complex inner surface, which could be described as corrugated, is arranged in such a way that it gives a very large surface. It is these corrugations – or 'villi,' as they are called – that cause most difficulty, because they become coated with catarrhal material. When this occurs they gradually become completely inactive and set up a resistance towards the passage of the foodstuffs through their walls into the blood and lymphatic streams.

This point is of great importance, and it is because of it that the two-day fast was advised at the beginning of the treatment. Nothing cleans up the bowel like fasting, especially if the fast is followed by an enema and a day on fruit. These combinations of fasting and fruit days have a tremendous effect on the assimilative powers, and once the patient is able to assimilate vegetables and fruits the supply of mineral salts to the blood can be greatly increased.

Now comes the study of the starchy foods. These are taken to supply heat and energy and, as stated above, have usually been taken too liberally by the person suffering from catarrhal deafness and head noises. It is rather an unpleasant duty to restrict the starches. This is naturally difficult in a country such as Britain, which is cold and damp for long periods, when the body craves for some stimulation and heat from the starchy foods. This is all admitted, but it should be remembered that we have set out to remove a certain set of symptoms and to create healthful conditions inside the body.

STARCH DIGESTION

Experience teaches that catarrhal deafness is due largely to the consuming of too much milk and too many starchy foods, together with poor lymphatic circulation. It is my duty to warn sufferers against these foods and liquids. Commonly it is found that starch is taken at nearly every meal, but in this treatment an attempt will be made to restrict it to one meal. Starch digestion starts in the mouth and is continued in the duodenum and small bowel. It is a type of digestion which is rather tricky, and to make the operation more simple it is desirable to take all the daily starches at one meal.

This meal can be chosen to suit the person, but is best taken in the evening. The starches advised are potatoes, wholewheat products and cereals, and they are much more beneficial when they are compost grown and not forced by artificial manures. Potatoes are best baked in their jackets or steamed, because important minerals lie just beneath the skin. Wholewheat products are also good starches, but it is wise to seek variety in this type of food because by doing so the whole of the digestive tract connected with starch assimilation is re-educated.

It would be falling into a digestive error if we kept to the one type of wholewheat all the time, and that is why this point is stressed. Practically any food except acid fruit can be taken with starch. Butter combines well, as do other fats such as margarine, olive oil and nut cream. Vegetables of all kinds and the dried fruits are also suitable combinations with the starchy food, and there is no reason why any mixture of these suitable starchy foods should not be taken.

The next class of food is the proteins. These are fish, eggs, cheese, meat of all kinds, milk, peas, beans, lentils and nuts. They are the building foods and are essential to health in youth, to a lesser degree in middle age and in still smaller amounts in old age. It is usually thought by dietitians that too many proteins are found in the diet of people who have reached middle or old age, and it is suspected that these foods, taken in excess, contribute to blood, heart, liver and kidney ailments. Certainly all these troubles are relieved by a reduction in protein food.

REDUCED PROTEIN INTAKE

This finding does ıot directly apply in the case of the person suffering from catarrhal deafness, but if one protein only is taken each day then the liver will be relieved of strain. This organ is associated with blood cleansing and has a great deal of work to do in the cure of deafness. To adhere to one protein only each day is difficult to accomplish, perhaps, because a meal seems to have something lacking if a protein is not taken; but if the person who is following this diet will carry on over the first few weeks with a reduced protein intake, the habit will be broken. A meal without protein is not so satisfying, but it is more health giving. Still, there is usually not so much need to pay a great deal of attention to the proteins in this trouble. Take the best of them in limited quantities, and introduce them in the mixtures arranged in the diet sheet.

Liquid in the diet always presents a problem, because there are some people who feel they must drink and others who are not thirsty. It all depends on the diet, type of work and build of the person. It suffices to state that liquids should, generally speaking, be reduced in people who are stout. Liquids are definitely detrimental in cases of high blood pressure and dropsy, but these conditions are outside the scope of this book. The best plan is to take liquid only when thirsty and to remember that tea, coffee, wines, spirits and alcohol are definitely harmful. Milk must be regarded as completely unsuitable. It will cause catarrh in nearly all circumstances, and when the catarrh is located in such a vital organ as the ear the milk must be stopped immediately. The same applies to all foods made with milk. Other foods that are also harmful are all white flour products, including bread, pastry, cakes, scones and all foods make from patent flours, including all milk puddings. These foods are lacking in the balanced mineral salts and vitamins, and they tend to extract from the system the salts that normally should be supplied in food. In other words, when a person takes unbalanced foods the store of minerals in the body is reduced, because the system leeches its minerals from the store unnecessarily; indeed, cases have occurred in which the body has drawn its minerals direct from the bones.

BUILD ON WHOLEWHEAT

This point is appreciated by flour manufacturers, and in their advertisements for white flour it is stated that valuable salts have been reintroduced after milling. A moment's thought will show that it is impossible to introduce these salts in the same proportion and in the same character as they were in the natural grains. Build your diet on wholewheat, and do not be tempted to take any food because it is specifically stated that this food has been reinforced in any way. Good food, grown on healthy, compost-manured soil, does not require any reinforcement, and in itself is capable of supplying everything that the body requires. If, however, it is impossible to gain the benefit of wholewheat products, then the addition of wheat germ in the form of a health food supplement is advised. Wheat germ is actually the vital part of the wheat and can be used to replace substances lost in milling.

Other substances that come within the category of those detrimental to health are: condiments, preserves, especially preserves that contain commercial sugar, foods containing flavourings and fillers of all kinds, fried and greasy foods, excessive salt and food containing salt, medicines that have some form of salt as a base. This is especially found in laxatives, and even those can be harmful in cases of catarrhal deafness.

5. The Diet

IT IS NATURALLY difficult in the compass of a small book to explain a diet suitable for everyone suffering from this trouble, and the diet outlined must be regarded as a general one. In the everyday practice of Nature Cure, the diets are changed frequently to suit the varying conditions through which the patients are passing, because it is found that many idiosyncrasies prevent them from keeping to set diets. The reader should however, if he is not under naturopathic supervision, give this treatment a fair chance and only make changes when foods are definitely unsuitable.

This diet has proved successful in many cases of catarrhal deafness, but the final diet must never include foods that have been described here as detrimental. It is, of course, possible that certain food combinations may not agree. If this is so they should be stopped for a few days, then tried again, because it is usually found that as the blood changes, the various food combinations become more suitable to the patient. When it is found that a certain food disagrees, then discontinue it for a week. During this time the system will have changed, and then the food should be tried again when it will often be found that it can be tolerated.

Each day on this diet means that the bloodstream is changing for the better, becoming more positive and health-giving. It also means that the impurities within your body are being taken right through the system and are being delivered at the eliminating organs. If these organs are working efficiently (this will be discussed in a later chapter) it will be found that the degree of health is increasing each day. This does not mean that no difficulties will arise. Real health is seldom static. Each day the body is attempting, by every means in its power, to eliminate impurities, to assimilate the food it requires, and such undertakings cannot take place without upset.

This is a tried and proved system of healing, and it can be practised with complete faith. Always believe that the body is doing the correct thing, and develop all efforts along the lines of helping and never hindering it. That is to say, if you don't feel well and have lost appetite, then don't eat. If your mouth is dry, then don't eat. If you are nervously upset or worried in any way, then don't eat. Beware of false hunger, because often food is taken when there is no real desire, and in these circumstances harm is often done to the system. So important is the above that it is best set down in the form of food rules.

Rule One. Never eat when not hungry. The habit in this country of eating at mealtimes, instead of when we are actually hungry, is very dangerous, and often food is taken when our stomach and digestive organs are not in a fit condition to deal with it. Real compelling hunger is the best appetizer, and the appetite should never be tempted in any false way. If our body requires food, then hunger arises; if hunger is absent, then all food should be stopped until it returns. A feeling of slight hunger at all times is a good sign.

Rule Two. The second rule is never to eat when emotionally upset – that is, if worried or nervously tense in any way. There may, in these circumstances, be a desire for food, but it is always abnormal and is often followed by gastric upset. So if emotionally upset, tensed, worried, then avoid food and liquid. Ensure relaxation before any food is taken, and even then take very small quantities.

Rule Three. Food that is in any way distasteful should be avoided. Under social obligations people are often forced to take food that is not suitable. The reader of this book, who is trying to cure a special condition, should avoid the taking of substances that are not to taste, and, although this may cause some disagreeableness, it is well worth taking a stand against indiscriminate eating.

Rule Four. The fourth rule in our study of when food should be taken is never to eat when tired. Digestion is a chemical, physical and nervous process, and as such it demands a considerable amount of physical energy. When tired, a normal physical reaction is not obtained, and the digestion of the food is often very much impaired. Food taken then is often so poorly digested that it enters the system in an unfinished state and readily gives rise to catarrhal debris.

Rule Five. Never eat when the mouth is dry. This does not mean the normal thirst that follows exertion on a hot day, but rather the abnormal heated condition that comes into the mouth when there is fever present or the dry heat that comes when the system is very much upset emotionally. In fevers or in high emotion the mouth becomes very dry, and it is our duty to obey this sign and avoid food. When the digestive system is ready for food, the gastric juices flow freely and the mouth is moist. Food taken at this time means that a proper intermixing of the digestive juices is obtained and assimilation is likely to be efficient.

Some time has been taken to stress these points because they are very important, and a spendidly balanced, wholesome diet can be spoiled by taking food under conditions that do not warrant complete digestion. It must be remembered that the formation of catarrhal material within our system depends on many things, but primarily it arises from the incomplete digestion of starchy foods. If these are not fully utilized by the body, then the amount left tends to become catarrh.

ON RISING

It is always advisable when there is catarrh in the system to take a glass of water each morning on rising. Now this glass of water should be according to desire, and naturally this will vary from day to day. If one day cold water is desired it does not follow that it will be suitable each morning; the next morning warm water may appeal more. But hot or cold, it is good treatment to introduce some water into the digestive tract before any solid food is taken. It is also often useful to add some lemon juice with this water. It need not be a large amount; a teaspoonful or even ten drops are quite sufficient. If this juice is suitable and does not cause a great deal of digestive upset, then it will aid greatly in neutralizing and removing the catarrhal material.

Taking such an acid fruit juice is not advised when there is already present an acid condition such as rheumatism, arthritis, skin trouble or gastric or duodenal ulceration. The reason for this is not hard to seek. The body is already acid, and adding another acid only drains the alkaline salts which are already in reduced amounts. In such cases, as the treatment progresses, it will often be found that this juice can then be taken, but as a general rule it should be avoided until any acid condition has been removed. If the lemon juice causes digestive acidity it should be stopped in the meantime.

BREAKFAST

The breakfast for the catarrhal deaf patient should vary considerably from that of a person on normal diet. Best of all is the fresh acid fruit diet – that is, a meal consisting of the following fruits when in season: apples, oranges, grapefruit, grapes, pears, all kinds of berries and juices such as apple, lemon, orange, grape and pineapple. These fruits can be taken in any quantity to suit the taste. They are very energetic cleansers, and if the digestion is strong enough they will bring about invigoration of the blood and lymphatic streams and will expel many impurities from the body. The fruit juice can be obtained in bottled form.

The acid fruits are necessary for the cure of this condition. They do not supply any great food value, but they abound in vitamins and mineral salts, which are needed by people with poor hearing. The acid fruit breakfast, however, is not a satisfying one, and most patients rise from the table feeling that they have not had enough to eat. This is quite a natural feeling, and it should be expected. A person leaving the table in such a state has not overloaded the digestive system and is able to deal readily and easily with the foods that have been introduced.

The people who are already very acidic will have extreme difficulty in digesting these fruits, and in some cases it is an impossibility. This viewpoint often changes within a few weeks, when it will be common to find that the person who could not deal digestively with any acid fruit is able to take it in small amounts. This is a very important finding which has already been stressed. It will be easily understood that as the chemistry of the blood changes, the power to deal with the various foods also changes. When, however, the acid fruit breakfast cannot be taken, the breakfast should be based on the following: wholewheat cereal or muesli added to soaked and simmered prunes, figs or raisins or stewed apples or pears.

It will be noticed that no milk is advised; instead the cereal should be placed in the juice of the fruit. This makes an ideal laxative, and if there is any trouble with constipation this is perhaps more efficacious than the ordinary breakfast, which is often not corrective in constipation. In cases of chronic constipation, crude black molasses can be added to the cereal.

With this type of breakfast it is also permissible to have some starch in the form of thin wholewheat toast, rye crispbread and one brown digestive biscuit. Vegetable extracts are allowed as liquids, but in most cases it is preferable that the meal should be taken as dry as possible, to ensure mastication. This meal is actually a mixture of starch and fruit, and although the acid fruits form the ideal breakfast it will usually be found that the mixture of dried fruit and starches will be much more suitable digestively. The reader must understand, however, that the acid fruit breakfast is always the most helpful, and it should be taken whenever possible.

FORENOON

During the forenoon, if there is any hunger, suitable fruit should be taken in any quantity and in any mixture. If it is found that this fruit upsets the appetite or causes digestive acidity, naturally it should be stopped.

SECOND MEAL

This can be described as the protein meal, and it is better to take one form of protein and not mix several proteins, to make digestion simple.

Start the meal with vegetable soup, provided a mixture of fluid and solid does not cause acidity.

Then take cheese or egg protein (lightly cooked) or a vegetarian dish made with peas, beans, lentils or nuts. All these proteins are good and are preferable to flesh or fish.

With the proteins take steamed or casseroled vegetables but no potatoes. A mixture of protein and starch tends to create a false appetite.

Dessert: fruit, including all forms of berries, apples, oranges, pears, tinned pineapple or the dried fruit such as prunes, figs or raisins.

No other food or liquid.

AFTERNOON

One cup of weak China tea may be taken if desired.

THIRD MEAL

This meal should be mainly starch and vegetables.

If there is actual thirst, vegetable soup may be taken again.

A large mixed salad, including lettuce, tomato, watercress, celery, cucumber, grated carrot or turnip, mustard and cress, endive, syboes, grated onions, beetroot, fruit such as chopped or grated apples, pears, oranges, dates, raisins, figs, bananas, tinned or fresh pineapple, appricots, peaches. Honey and lemon juice or olive oil and lemons as dressing.

Potatoes. Wholewheat bread or scone, rye crispbread or brown digestive biscuit. Honey, butter.

It will be noticed that no protein foods are advised at this meal, but a person with good digestive powers can occasionally take a small helping of cheese, egg or grated nuts without any upset.

If fluid is required with this meal, then it should be limited to weak china tea, maté tea, or vegetable extracts.

SUPPER
Fruit of any kind is allowed. No fluid.

6.
Elimination

THE FOREGOING DIET has been arranged with certain factors in mind, and one of these is that such a diet aids the elimination of impurities from the body. The meals given are so arranged that there is no clogging of the various organs that have as their function, or part of their function, the removal of food debris. Now the reader may be puzzled about this statement, because it seems peculiar that debris should be introduced into the body; yet every food and nearly every liquid contains substances which are extraneous to the body's economy.

Our bodies are so designed that they can deal adequately with a reasonable amount of impurity, and every minute of the day the eliminating organs are working and throwing this out. If these special organs are not working correctly, the amount of impurity rises until it is abnormal and, in the case of catarrhal deafness, until some has been lodged in and around the hearing apparatus. In this chapter the work of the organs of elimination will be explained more fully to enable the reader to realize why the diet has been built in a certain manner.

The organs of elimination are the kidneys, lungs, bowel and skin, and they will be dealt with in that order.

THE KIDNEYS

The kidneys deal mainly with impurities such as urea, uric acid and certain salts. These arise from the digestion of protein foods (meat, fish, fowl, peas, beans, lentils, milk), and it is interesting to note that the kidneys of a vegetarian have normally to do only half the work of the kidneys of a meat eater. This does not, of course, mean that everyone suffering from catarrhal deafness requires to become a vegetarian, but if there are definite signs of kidney distress then this course is advisable. The signs of kidney trouble are usually easily recognizable and include swelling of the loose tissues of the ankles, abdomen and below the eyes, headache, visual disturbances, changes in the blood pressure and great tiredness. If this condition becomes very severe, certain forms of fits may arise and bladder changes are noticeable.

If these symptoms accompany or are even evident in minor degree in the case of catarrhal deafness, it is advisable to study the diet and make little changes, such as stopping flesh protein and reducing the amount of liquid. This advice may seem peculiar, because most physicians are inclined to increase the amount of liquid when there is kidney distress. It has been found, however, that such a course only gives the kidneys more work to do, and the dry diet is usually the best course.

Notice that I have said that these changes arc only required when there are definite signs of kidney trouble. The diet as arranged will deal adequately with most conditions of kidney disturbances of a minor nature. If there is a definite obstruction of elimination through the kidneys, then the use of the cold compress, which will be described in the chapter on local treatments, is advisable. This compress should be worn at night and should be used four times weekly, provided, of course, that the reaction is sufficient. Tea, coffee, alcohol, aerated waters and excessive salting of foods are dangerous to the kidneys.

THE LUNGS

It will be noted that the amount of starch in the diet is severely limited. This has the effect of greatly relieving the strain on the lungs, which have the duty of removing carbonic acid gas from the body and introducing oxygen. When the diet is low in milk and starch it is found that there is practically an immediate reaction on the lungs; they become much clearer, and a deeper inhalation can be obtained with less effort. This is very important, and it shows how one part of the body can be particularly affected by careful dieting. At the same time it will be easily understood that the lungs can be re-educated by practising deep-breathing exercises, and to the earnest reader I would advocate that a system be laid down which should be practised daily.

Deep breathing is only natural on exertion, and when performed as an exercise it must be artificial in some degree, but the end result can be very beneficial. Deep breathing is especially beneficial in catarrhal deafness, because it creates movement in the upper part of the chest and aids the drainage of the tissues round the ears. Here are three breathing exercises that will be of benefit.

EXERCISE ONE: Stand erect with the arms by the side. Take a deep breath, drawing the air in slowly through the nostrils and allowing the chest, by the expansion of the lungs, to move upwards and outwards. The main mistake in this exercise is to move the chest wall by muscular effort. This is naturally wrong because the intake of air should force the chest into its new position. When this position is reached, hold the breath for a few seconds and then exhale slowly through the nose or mouth, according to preference, pressing the ribs downwards and inwards with the hands and bending the body forward to aid the expulsion. This exercise should be practised twenty times daily. A slight increase in the chest expansion is always desirable, but what is more helpful is the obtaining of rib movement.

EXERCISE TWO: Stand erect with the hands at the sides, slowly inhale a full breath through the nostrils, at the same time bending to the right, thus reducing the capacity of the right lung. From this position bend slowly to left, exhaling until the limit of movement is achieved. This compresses the left lung. Continue in this way for ten movements, then change the system of breathing, breathing in as you bend to the left and out as you bend to the right. This ensures that both lungs are used.

EXERCISE THREE: Lie on the back with the arms by the sides. Take a deep breath, and fill the chest until the diaphragm is forced downwards and the abdomen rises. Hold for a few seconds and then exhale, pulling the abdomen inwards and towards the chest. This valuable exercise should be performed ten times. It is a movement that is frequently practised incorrectly, and I advise the reader to imagine the air going in through the lung and forcing the diaphragm downwards and forcing the abdominal wall upwards. Once this imaginary idea is gained, the movement becomes very simple.

THE BOWEL

The third organ of elimination is the bowel, and generally this is regarded by lay people as the most important. This is not correct, however; the other organs with eliminative function are just as important, if not more so. The bowel receives the partially digested foodstuff and passes it downwards until nothing but unwanted food is contained in the large bowel. As this unwanted food has never actually been taken into the tissues of the body, what is termed elimination of bodily waste is really only the passing of food that has not been used. Admittedly there is a certain amount of elimination through the actual wall of the bowel, but this does not compare with that from the kidneys or from the skin. So the bowel is actually a passage through the body, and if it is supplied with roughage it will generally look after itself.

It will usually be found that the bowel assumes a different rhythm when a balanced diet is followed, and even the end-products of such a dietary are harmless. Rhythm naturally varies with each person, and it is impossible to say what is really normal for that person; but if a good diet is followed and the exercise of the person is adequate, the bowel will set up its own rhythm and will work when it requires to do so. It should never be forced in any way, and the taking of laxatives, especially salt in any form, is not advised, because this can be a factor in the formation of catarrh.

If laxatives are required at all, and this should be very seldom, those of the herbal variety are best. True constipation is not so common as is supposed, and the patient must be certain that he or she is suffering in this way before an attempt is made to cure the condition. The signs of constipation are excessive tiredness, lack of appetite, coated tongue, greasy skin with outbreaks and a general feeling of ill-health, accompanied, of course, by a peculiar bowel rhythm, several days passing before a movement is obtained.

When all these signs are present, steps must be taken to deal with constipation. On the other hand, if a person feels well and looks well and none of the signs of constipation are apparent, any kind of bowel rhythm may be normal and need not cause any worry. It is possible for the bowel to move even every third day and the person still not be constipated.

This is important, because most people worry a great deal about constipation, and some make themselves feel ill because the bowel is not moving daily or even twice daily. This is absolutely wrong, and once it is recognized that the bowel rhythm is variable with each person, there will come some emotional relief.

THE SKIN

The last organ of elimination, the skin, is most important. When it is working effectively a great deal of strain is removed from the other organs that have this function. The skin, the largest of the eliminating organs, passes to the outside several pints of invisible perspiration daily, and also expresses various oily matters that are not helpful to the body.

The skin is greatly aided in its work when the sugary starches and sugars, so common in the ordinary diet, are reduced. Everyone who suffers from a poor complexion should reduce the starches and sugars, and a definite improvement will soon show in the condition of their skin. The diet advised, low in starch and fairly low in sugars, will bring about some relief to an overworked skin, but this tissue can be further stimulated by friction rubbing with a rough towel or flesh gloves or, better still, by rubbing with the hands. Dip the hands in cold water and apply to the skin, rubbing as vigorously as possible, and continue in this way, applying cold water all the time. This is a most invigorating treatment which thins the skin and makes the elimination of impurities a very much easier business.

Sun-ray, especially sun-ray combined with massage, is also a most helpful measure for retoning the skin and should be taken by everyone who finds that the skin is thick and unhealthy. Notice that it has been stated that an unhealthy skin is thick. The healthy skin should be dry and thin; that is, it can be raised from the underlying tissues fairly easily.

THINK BEFORE YOU EAT

It will now be seen that our diet, rich in mineral salts and vitamins, low in starch and protein, and with the complete cessation of milk and milk products, is a most helpful one for the elimination of impurities already within the system.

The lungs are helped by a reduction of starch and certain forms of sugar. The kidneys are aided by the reduction of tea, coffee and certain proteins, especially those that are fried. The bowel is helped by the introduction of rougher food and also by the stoppage of milky starches. The skin is invigorated by a reduction in sugar foods. These are all very helpful aids to the treatment, and they make the cleansing of the body much easier. Only a few weeks will elapse before this cleansing is appreciated, and the person undergoing the cure will feel lighter and better in every way.

This progress from ill-health towards health is gradual, but it can be accelerated if the organs of elimination and their action are always kept in mind. Before you eat something and before you do something – think. Ask yourself whether it can possibly delay elimination; and if by any means it can, it should be avoided. The body is very finely balanced in most cases, and there seems to be only a hair's breadth between the condition of acidity and alkalinity.

7. Local Treatment

THE READER WILL naturally be anxious to know what can be done locally to increase the actual healing powers, but it must be remembered that the initial cause of deafness is the formation of catarrh within the body. The foregoing treatment is the most important, and without it local measures will not be effective.

Two main changes in the body have been achieved. The diet has been so re-designed that very little catarrhal-forming food is introduced, the eliminative part of the body has been stimulated and the amount of impurity within the body reduced. In other words, the treatment outlined will have created favourable conditions, and if it has been conducted faithfully, the chances of removing this troublesome condition are very much enhanced.

In practice it is found that months may elapse, depending on the condition of the patient, before actual improvement is noticed, although a quick result is obtained every now and then. Six months is the usual period required by the body to get its curative efforts to the effective stage. This may, at first sight, appear a long time, but it must be remembered that this is a cure, not merely a method of suppression. The causes of deafness are being removed, not pushed deeper into the system, as is so often done in other treatments.

It must also be mentioned that it is never wise to attempt local treatment before the general constitutional measures outlined have been carefully followed. If this is not the case, then the local treatments about to be explained are not suitable; indeed, they can be definitely harmful, because treatment may bring impurities to the ear and a much worse condition may be created.

CONSULTATION

Very little is done by medical practitioners to cure catarrhal deafness. The sufferer is usually advised to apply medicated drops, protect the eardrums from chill and perform the daily gargle. Ear specialists, if these are consulted, often inflate the eustachian tubes, but otherwise the treatment is the same. If these practitioners actually appreciated the real cause of the trouble, they would set about the cure in very much the same manner as outlined in this book.

Naturally, for local treatment, professional advice is the most effective, and whenever possible anyone who suffers from catarrhal deafness should consult a trained naturopath. These practitioners are to be found in most large towns, although they are not so numerous as medical practitioners. This course is advised because in many cases of catarrhal deafness there is a lesion of the spinal bones in the neck.

These bones are relatively fine in structure, and because of their position they are commonly displaced. When this occurs it is possible that the nerves that emerge from between the bones are affected in some way, and very frequently the entire lymphatic drainage of the face is choked.

Poor drainage of the face and of the tissues near the face, including the ears, plus catarrh, can lead to deafness and head noises. It is for this reason that consultation with an osteopath is advised. These men are specially trained in spinal diagnosis and in the manipulative treatments that are so effective in correcting any spinal lesion.

When dislocation or lesion is mentioned, these terms are meant to cover any condition in which the spinal bones are not in their correct position. Lesion by itself seems to be rather a fearsome word, but it does not necessarily mean that great force has been used to displace a bone, but rather that one, two or three of the bones are slightly out of their normal position. This may not cause any pain, but the twisting of the muscles and ligaments nearby results in a nipping of the nerve. There are few cases of actual bony pressure on the nerve itself.

Whenever any twisting of the muscles and ligaments occurs,

the common accompaniment is tension. This itself can cause some pressure on the nerves leading from the neck and can be one of the factors in catarrhal deafness. Neck lesions are so common in this trouble that very few cases examined are found without such a condition.

The cause of poor circulation in the face area need not be an actual lesion of the spinal bones but may arise from clumps or clusters of rheumatic deposits on or near one of these bones. This acidic accumulation effects the nerves leading from the part, and it is often possible to feel these clusters with the fingers; here pressure is usually, but not always, painful. Trained manipulation combined with soft tissue massage will ease up this type of trouble very quickly, but in certain chronic cases heat treatment with prolonged massage may be required before the pressure is removed.

If it is not possible to obtain the services of a trained naturopath or osteopath, a physiotherapist should be consulted and asked if he can find anything wrong with the neck bones or muscles. In most cases the tension is readily discovered, and massage and radiant heat can be most helpful. This is naturally not so effective as manipulation, but it can be of use in reducing the more simple lesions.

The value of a diagnosis of the condition of the spine at the neck area has been considerably detailed, but it is worth while for any person suffering from this illness to go out of his way to get advice on this aspect. Exercises and water treatments outlined later in this book are extremely valuable, but professional examination of this method of manipulative treatment is always the best way of attacking the trouble.

Once the neck has been examined, and if any difficulties have been discovered and corrected, other local measures can be studied. If, however, it is impossible to obtain professional advice, the simple measures about to be explained should be tried out and professional advice sought at a later date.

REMOVAL OF WAX

These methods can be practised in the privacy of the home

without anyone else in the household knowing that something is being done to aid the deafness. In the first case, all wax of an excessive nature should be removed from the ears. When a person is in a catarrhal state it is very common indeed to find that wax is formed readily, and this is one of the reasons for the rapid increase in loss of hearing. If the ears can be syringed by a local practitioner, so much the better, but it is always advisable to soften the wax beforehand by putting in a few drops of almond oil or a mixture of almond oil and hydrogen peroxide. This should be allowed to work through the wax for a few days and then the physician should be asked to syringe the ear. Occasional syringing, say once every second year, is not harmful; but if it has to be done more frequently, say every six months, there is a tendency that the drum of the ear may become affected, and if it is at all weak, there is also a danger of perforation.

It is most unnatural to direct a violent jet of water against the ear drum, so it is always advisable to soften the wax gradually with almond oil and to work a long finger of cotton wool into the ear and patiently remove the wax. This treatment, if carried out every night for a time, will gradually result in most of the wax being removed, and the body, especially during the sleeping hours, will bring away any remnants of wax which still persist.

In this way the external meatus can be cleaned, and there is no danger, provided only a finger of cotton wool is used, of harming the drum. If, however, there is a very large core of wax after the initial soft wax has been removed, a little oil should be introduced each night for a week, and all the time the hard core of wax should be reduced by using the cotton wool. This may not result in the removal of very hardened wax, and this should be softened as much as possible before the physician, skilled in the use of the syringe, should be contacted.

Many people attempt to use a small syringe themselves but this is quite a dangerous method and is not at all advisable. It is far better to seek a physician or a naturopath to do this part of the cure. When this wax is removed it is quite common to find that the ear feels rather raw, and there may be a perceptible increase in the degree of hearing. Usually, however, in catarrhal deafness, most of the trouble lies on the other side of the drum, and until now we are only ensuring that the external meatus is completely clear.

GARGLING

Internally there is not a great deal to be done, because it is naturally difficult to reach this part of the mechanism; but we can do quite a lot to equalize the pressure on the outside of the ear drum with the pressure on the inside. First of all, there is great benefit in gargling. Each morning take a glass of hot water and gargle as deeply in the throat as possible. This will relax the throat and will often bring away an amount of catarrh from the eustachian tubes. These tubes run from the mouth into the inner side of the ear, and it is through them that much catarrh can be removed. If this is attempted for a few mornings, and no immediate result is shown, the amount of water should be increased, up to one pint; then it will usually be found that more and more catarrh is dropping into the back of the throat. This catarrhal material should, if possible, be coughed up, because if it is not, it will be retained in the digestive tract. If it is found that this catarrh is dropping into the digestive tract, a mild herbal laxative should be taken each day.

Cold water gargling is not advised, but it will be found, after a month on diet, that alternate hot and cold water gargling will be more useful in retoning the throat and the tubes leading from the throat to the ears. When doing this form of gargling always finish with the cold water, and if possible do it during the morning.

HOT AND COLD PACKS

Hot and cold packs applied to the area below the ear are also very useful in this condition. Use the hot pack as hot as the skin will stand for one minute, then apply the cold pack for half a minute. Continue in this way for ten minutes, and always finish with the cold pack. It is usually convenient to use the cold compress immediately after this alternate hot and cold packing, which should be done each evening.

COMPRESSING

The cold neck compress consists of a piece of linen some three inches broad which is soaked in cold water, wrung out and applied round the neck and fixed with a safety pin or tape. This is then covered with a piece of flannel or woollen material which should overlap the linen and completely cover it. With this neck compress a waist compress should also be worn, applied in the following manner. Take a piece of linen about eight inches broad, soak it in cold water, wring out, apply around the waist, and cover with flannel or woollen material. These compresses should heat up within ten minutes, this being ascertained by slipping the finger between the compress and the skin, when a moist heat will be found. If the compress does not heat it should be removed and tried again next night.

The waist and neck compresses should be worn five nights weekly if the reaction is good, and it is best to apply them before retiring and wear them all night. It is also of benefit if they are used just after the hot and cold packs have been applied.

THE HEAD STEAM BATH

In cases of catarrh it is found that many impurities are removed through the skin and scalp, and steam baths can then help the body in its cleansing. A steam bath once weekly is desirable in catarrhal deafness, and should be performed in the following manner:

First of all, thoroughly wash the hair and scalp, using plenty of warm water and a mild soap. Rinse thoroughly with warm water. Now fill up the wash-hand basin with very hot water and hold the face over the steam, covering the head with flannel until the face perspires vigorously. It often helps if a glass of hot fruit juice is taken just before the steaming. Finish this treatment by douching the face and head in cold water, thoroughly dry the hair by friction rubbing. Electric hair driers should not be used in this treatment.

These simple water treatments should be practised carefully and regularly. It will often be found that even after each treatment, some slight improvement in the hearing or the condition of the head noises is noticed. This usually disappears, but a gradual general improvement soon becomes evident.

HEAD COLD

If the sufferer is lucky enough to contract a head cold with a catarrhal discharge, this can be used as an eliminative effort, because much of the catarrh can then be removed from the ear passages. Care must be taken with this cold, and all water treatments should be stopped and a complete fast or a fruit fast commenced and continued until the cold clears up without treatment. This type of cold can be regarded as a cleansing crisis, and its value should be appreciated by all who suffer from catarrh.

8.
Some Cures

WHEN CATARRHAL DEAFNESS is being treated, the primary effort is directed at removing the catarrh; but owing to the position of the foreign matter, usually deep in the internal ear, this is not an easy matter. It requires a definite plan to be followed carefully over a somewhat lengthy period before results can be obtained. That some very good results are obtained there is no doubt, and the following cases will give some idea of the cures that can be wrought by this method, which, although simple, is most effective.

Case One. A middle-aged woman contracted a severe cold. At first this affected her chest, then gradually the throat became inflamed and, in spite of treatment, the infection spread into the ears. She became deaf, was very much troubled with head noises, and ultimately there arose a discharge from the left ear of yellow mucus. When this subsided, a week after it was first noticed, the hearing on this side was completely lost. After some time an ear specialist was consulted, and he tried various methods including inflation, the latter treatment being followed by slight improvement for some weeks, but the hearing was gradually lost again. Special drops were then applied to the ear, but these were of no avail and gradually the right ear became affected.

After this, many home cures were tried, but these made little difference and the physician reluctantly admitted that nothing else could be done.

The patient then submitted herself to a treatment very much the same as outlined in this book. Within three months there was a slight reduction in the head noises, and they changed in character from a loud buzzing and very irritating noise to one that was more or less a soft whistle, not so constant nor so irritating to the sufferer. About this time the patient confessed to the practitioner that she had given up all hope of ever hearing correctly again, but she was very pleased to have some relief from the head noises, which had been making her very short-tempered. She was instructed to continue the treatment with renewed vigour, and within two weeks she contracted a severe head cold. This was accompanied by an increase in intensity of the head noises, and there was a profuse discharge from the nasal passages and the general upset was quite severe. This, however, was the symptom for which the practitioner was waiting, and he arranged a special diet which was carefully followed by the patient. The cold took a similar course to the first one, which had caused all her trouble, but was more severe, and the throat gradually became very highly inflamed and would have been termed a quinsy throat by an allopathic practitioner.

In addition to the discharge from the nose there also arose a discharge from the ear, and once this started the throat became a little better. The discharge from the ear continued even after the cold was completely cured. The head noises were severe and the throat was inflamed, but these symptoms decreased in violence after the ears discharged, and gradually disappeared.

NORMAL HEARING RESTORED

The actual hearing was not much better after this upset, but professional hearing tests showed that the hearing had improved slightly and the patient was advised to continue the treatment. A month later another head cold appeared, not so severe as the previous colds, but still localized more or less in the head. It was treated by fasting and hot and cold compressing, and when it cleared up it was found that the patient's hearing was normal.

A report received five years after the completion of treatment indicated that the hearing was still normal. The above was an ideal case, but it proves that the methods, simple in many ways are very effective because they are based on allowing the natural healing properties of the body to effect a cure.

Case Two. This patient had a history of a nervous breakdown brought on by domestic upheaval. A spell of dizziness was followed by a severe attack of rheumatism which affected all his joints, but mainly those of the spine. He then lost all his hair, and his hearing became affected from this occurrence. Two months after the initial consultation he wrote that his rheumatism was less severe and that there was some improvement in his condition. He was able to reduce the amount of daily drugs until he was taking only one phenobarbitone tablet.

SINUS INFLAMMATION

Just after he had written this letter, without any warning whatsoever, he was attacked by a severe pain in the sinuses, which his local doctor had diagnosed as acute sinusitis. He was advised to try Nature Cure treatment. A complete fast, then a fruit fast, hot and cold applications to the face and a waist compress were the basic treatments, and after a few days it was found that all his symptoms had disappeared. A study of this patient's primary diagnosis showed that this sinus inflammation had occurred on various occasions, and it was then decided that it would be advisable to have his mouth X-rayed to see if there was any cause for this infection. The X-ray showed that there were two roots of teeth left in the upper jaw and that both of them were highly infected. These were extracted, and the patient called within a week of this slight operation and it was found then that the resonance of the voice was greatly improved. Much of the congestion had gone from his nasal passages, and he was able to breathe freely through his nostrils, a thing he had not been able to do for many years.

It would seem that in this case there had been this continual infection setting up a slight inflammation in the sinuses all the time and bringing about a condition of poor circulation to which the catarrhal deposits were drawn. Changes were then made in the treatment, mainly of a dietetic nature, and hearing tests were carried out each month. Within five months it was found that the hearing was practically normal, and so it remained, because this patient was examined regularly to ensure that the good result was maintained.

The reader may surmise that the presence of the decaying root in the jaw of this patient was the original cause, but actually the catarrhal impurity had been present for years and the infection of teeth only caused local congestion and impaired circulation.

HAIR RESTORED

The real causative factor was the catarrh, which had been brought about by poor diet. It is interesting also to note that the patient gradually recovered his hair growth. First of all, round about the time when his hearing was getting better, a fine, downy growth appeared on the scalp. This was stimulated by cold water and shaving, and soon proper growth was established. Now he has a good head of hair, although the colour seems to be slightly lighter than before. There is reason to believe that the hair was lost through the action of dandruff on the scalp, but connected with the nervous upset. Dandruff is a form of catarrh and as such can be treated internally as well as externally.

Case Three This was an elderly woman who had a history of catarrhal deafness for a period of a year, but who was now suffering from severe headaches, giddiness and accompanying symptoms which led to a diagnosis of an incurable condition from all standards. The patient was undoubtedly anaemic, and the treatment was first of all directed at this aspect, although the diet advised in this book would adequately cover such a contingency. Shortly after this, fasting was advised and the starch content of the diet reduced, with the usual emphasis laid on fresh fruit and vegetables, especially on the value of those having a red colouring, such as tomatoes, carrot, and beetroot. These foods stimulate blood formation. The patient was also slightly jaundiced, and this reacted quickly to the diet and she became very much younger-looking and fresher in every way, owing to the increased health in the liver area. She was not attending for actual manipulative treatment but was doing a number of carefully designed exercises, very much on the lines given in this book. These exercises could be termed the home manipulations, because they have very much the same effect as the actual manipulation conducted by the practitioner, although they take a much longer time to achieve their results. Exercising in this manner, carefully and systematically over a period, stretches the muscles to their fullest extent and allows bones which have been slightly misaligned to move back to their proper place.

CLEANSING BILIOUS ATTACK

Within a month the compression headache of this patient had disappeared, and although her deafness was not much better there was a reduction in the intensity of the head noises, so that she was again able to wear her hearing aid. This had been most uncomfortable, owing to the continued head noises and the occasional shrieking and buzzing that occurs with such instruments. The cleansing in this case came very suddenly, actually before it was expected, and it took the form of a bilious attack. The sickness was continuous for a day and the bowel was also active at the same time and much catarrhal material was passed in the stools. The patient appreciated an improvement in her hearing and she was able to hear a person speaking loud without her instrument. The head noises, however, although reduced in intensity, were still present, and soon they were again fairly troublesome. Exactly six weeks after the first attack of biliousness the patient had another. This was less severe, and again much catarrhal material was freed. The head noises, which seemed to increase in intensity just before the attack, were completely absent after it passed.

The hearing of this patient is still improving, and she does not use an instrument at all nowadays except when in a room with a number of people, when the hearing again falls, no doubt because of increased nervous tension.

9.
Head Noises

ALTHOUGH IN THIS book head noises have been treated as an allied condition to catarrhal deafness, it is also common to find that they can be present without any hearing trouble.

The condition of noise in the ear varies considerably with each person. In some cases it occurs only at specific times of the day, usually when the person is tired. In others it is common when the person becomes excited or emotionally strained in any way, and in still other cases it is present all the time, even if the person wakens during the night. The sounds heard vary considerably. A hissing like escaping steam is very common, a ringing like a bell or a loud buzzing are also usual forms, and again these sounds vary greatly in intensity. In some cases they get much louder when the patient is excited.

The effect of all this is gradually to bring about a great increase in nervous tension, and a person suffering from this type of illness, especially if of an excitable nature, becomes very easily irritated and tends to have fits of depression and anger.

There are several main causes of head noises, and although most of them are associated with catarrhal deafness of some form, there are others in which deafness does not complicate. In elderly people one of the most common causes of head noise is some hardening of the arteries, a condition called, medically, arterio-sclerosis. This is usually taken as a natural sign of increasing years, and it means that the elastic arteries, which expand and contract, according to the pumping of the heart, are becoming hardened and less mobile. There is a tendency for the arteries in the ear to become quickly affected, and the pumping of the heart is conveyed to the hearing mechanism and often is the noise causing the symptoms.

It is not, of course, possible in elderly people to reduce this tendency to any great degree, but it is possible to diminish artero-sclerosis and to keep it from progressing. The diet outlined in this book is an excellent basis for treating this trouble, if special attention is paid to the stoppage of tea, coffee and alcoholic liquors.

The protein foods are also dangerous in this condition, and they should be limited in quantity to one protein each day. A large amount of vegetables is required in this diet. These food changes, combined with the general treatment outlined in this book, will bring about a slow improvement in the condition and will reduce the intensity of the head noises.

Another cause of this trouble is very high blood pressure. This is a common accompaniment of bowel and kidney ailments, and in such cases the value of the cold waist compress cannot be overlooked. This compress should be applied, as already described, five nights weekly, provided, of course, that the reaction is good. It will bring about quite an appreciable reduction in the blood pressure within a few weeks.

DRY DIET

The diet for high blood pressure is a dry one, and the intake of liquid should be reduced so that only a little water, vegetable soup or fruit juice is taken daily. The proteins are also dangerous for this condition and must be kept to very small proportions. Rest, especially during the afternoon, is most helpful, and all emotional strain and vigorous physical exertion must be avoided until the blood pressure is at a lower level. It can be confidently expected, however, that a person wearing compresses and keeping to the diet outlined, especially when such diet is kept dry, will obtain quite a substantial reduction in the blood pressure.

This does not mean that every blood pressure can be brought back to normal. That is often impossible, owing to the state of the arteries, but in most cases it can be reduced from a dangerous level until it is possible for the person to get rid of the head noises. Low blood pressure – that is, a condition in which the highest pressure in the bloodstream, when the left ventricle of the heart is pumping, is below the normal – also causes head noises. This may actually be due to brain anaemia, a result of the low blood pressure, and in the upright position it is possible that the blood does not circulate freely through the brain area.

DIET FOR LOW BLOOD PRESSURE

Although this condition is not usually so serious as high blood pressure, it is often more difficult to eradicate. A general building diet is required, and the diet should be based on the lines outlined in this book. Two proteins – that is, two helpings of nuts, eggs, cheese, peas, beans, lentils, or any mixture of these proteins – can be taken daily. Vegetable soup is very helpful, and if there is no catarrh the milk diet can be used with advantage. Compressing is usually not required in these cases, but rest, combined with a moderate scheme of exercise, including plenty of deep breathing, is indicated.

Do not expect, however, that the blood pressure will rise rapidly. When a person has reached the stage in which the blood pressure is very low, it will take months before the body can recover sufficiently to raise the pressure again. People who talk rather glibly about blood pressure do not appreciate the difficulties in restoring it to normal. Certainly drug treatment can appear to be very beneficial, but most drugs work on the principle of contracting the arteries and the final result can be detrimental.

In Nature Cure, with the low protein and low starch diet, it is common to find that the blood pressure is below normal, and this may cause some mental distress. Actually, there is nothing to worry about, because the person with a slightly low blood pressure – that is, a few points below normal – has a much better chance of survival than the person with a high pressure. There is much less strain on the arteries and veins. The kidneys are not overworked, and although the person may lead a quieter life, perhaps – that is, there is not the same artificial stimulation as with the higher blood pressure – he certainly will live a much longer one, and the danger of cerebral haemorrhage will be much reduced. High blood pressure forces the heart to work against a resistance that finally strains this organ and makes the incident of heart disease very common. The same condition strains the arteries and is nearly always associated with some form of arterio-sclerosis.

These are very interesting points, and although the general treatment outlined for the catarrhal deafness again comes into practice in most of these cases, the slight difference in the dry and fluid diets should be noted. The fluid diet is very valuable in low blood pressure.

IMPURE FOODS

One of the very common causes of head noises, and one that is very seldom stressed in any writings on this subject, is the presence within the food of some impurity. Now this impurity is directly introduced into the bloodstream from the bowel, and it often travels to one of the end arteries, where it can cause irritation by its very presence. Salicylic acid is the most common offender, and it is used in many substances, especially in tinned food and in certain milk treatments. This is one of the reasons why tinned foods are not advised, except perhaps tinned pineapple, which is fairly free of impurity, and also why milk is not included in our diet. These things are difficult to discover, and it is only by chemical investigation that it is appreciated that the fillers, sparers, fat expanders and other chemicals introduced to preserve food can be harmful to our make-up.

Drugs, especially those of the quinine group, have an effect on head noises, and even the excessive use of aspirins can be a cause. Whenever possible, make your own bread and take food that is untreated in any way. You are then doing as much as you possibly can to prevent the entrance into the body of impure substances. We are very much at sea with regard to this chemicalization, and it is difficult even for a person studying food chemistry to make decisions and avoidance of all suspect food is the best way of ensuring health.

HAIR DYES ARE DANGEROUS

Hair dyes of all kinds are strongly advised against if there is any head noise. These substances definitely affect the hearing adversely, and although it is again difficult to determine whether this is a direct or indirect result, experience proves that their use is detrimental to the scalp and arterial and nervous systems. Many women who continually dye their hair gradually have trouble with headaches, skin ailments, hearing difficulties and head noises. This is because the scalp is frequently used by the body as an eliminative tissue, and it is most effective if kept clean, washed regularly and brushed in the ordinary way.

The application of hair oil may be slightly suppressive, but the use of dyes of any kind is definitely dangerous. The cleansing powers of the body are much reduced by their use, with the result that the impurities which were being pushed through the scalp then become submerged in the lower of innermost layers and affect the brain tissues and the apparatus of hearing. There is no actual benefit in undergoing this treatment if the hair is going to be continually dyed. This one factor can cause all the trouble, and the person who has been dyeing his or her hair will find an appreciable relief immediately dyeing is stopped and replaced only by general hair hygiene.

Again it must be understood that many sweets contain dyes and chemicals which can affect the nervous system and may cause head noises. These must be stopped, and whenever possible the sugar required in the diet should be obtained from honey and the other natural sweet foods.

These are the main factors in the other types of head noises, but basically the treatment is the same as that for catarrhal deafness; and the person who carries out such a treatment and adds any of the hints given in this chapter will be certain of speeding the cure.